# Kama Sutra

Dearest Steph —
may your married
life be full of romance
... etc.

Love :
Best wishes —
Lynn

*First HarperCollins Edition 1993*

*LC 92-56111*

*ISBN 0-06-250831-8*

*93 94 95 96 97 XXX 10 9 8 7 6 5 4 3 2 1*

*WARNING: With the prevalence of AIDS and other sexually*
*transmitted diseases, if you do not practice safe sex you*
*are risking your life and your partner's life.*

# KAMA SUTRA

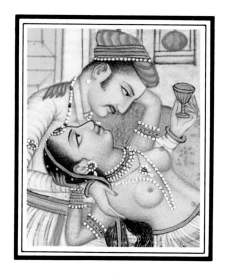

HarperSanFrancisco

*A Division of* HarperCollins*Publishers*

# INTRODUCTION

The Kama Sutra is one of the great books of the world. It was written in Benares nearly two thousand years ago by the elderly sage Vatsyayana. He had gone to the sacred city on the Ganges to end his days and he regarded the composition of the work as a religious duty. In Hinduism sex is holy and making love is a sacrament - a re-enactment of the divine union of the god and goddess.

Although it is the greatest of the Hindu love manuals, Kama Sutra is part of a continuous tradition. Vatsyayana drew upon a vast body of erotology which had accumulated over earlier centuries, choosing what he wanted and adding comments of his own. Later, his own work was treated in much the same way by the writers of the Indian Middle Ages. The text in this present book is taken mainly from the translation of Kama Sutra commissioned and edited by Sir Richard Burton and F.F. Arbuthnot, but the extracts from Vatsyayana's famous sixty-four - the chapter dealing with sex - have been augmented by new translations from the medieval love texts which took Kama Sutra as their model. This has been done to reflect the breadth and variety of Indian love teachings and to encourage those who are new to these wonderful books to read not only the complete, unabridged Kama Sutra, but also Ananga-Ranga and Koka Shastra which are available in translation.

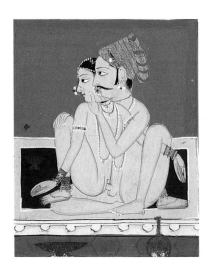

*Hindu love manuals are full of advice at a practical level - although the positions described in some of them are practical only for the double-jointed or for professional gymnasts - but there is a far more important message common to all the teachings. That is that sex is not sinful but beautiful, and that men and women are eternally complementary and equal. The corollary is that any system which denies those truths, denies life.*

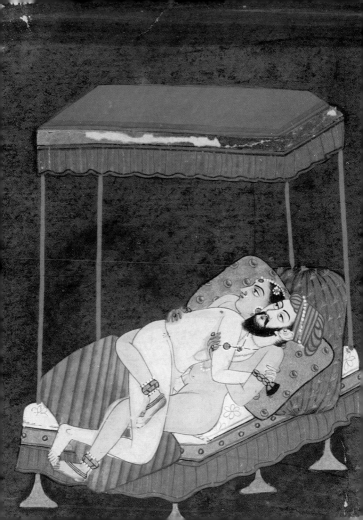

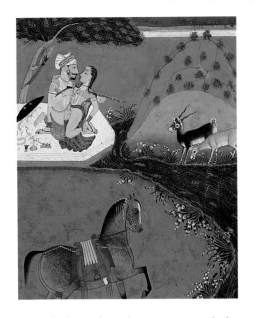

*Kama is to be learnt from the* Kama Sutra *which means simply the 'Science of Love'.*

*Kama is the enjoyment of appropriate objects by the five senses of hearing, feeling, seeing, tasting and smelling - assisted by the mind together with the soul*

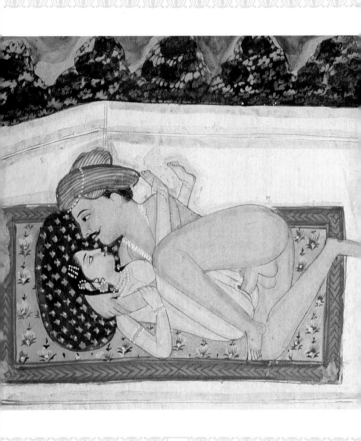

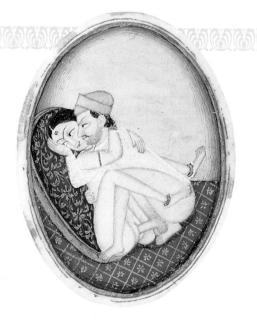

That part of the Kama Sutra *which deals with sexual union is called the 'sixty-four'. A man skilled in the sixty-four is looked upon with love by his own wife, by the wives of others, and by courtesans.*

*If a wife becomes separated from her husband, and falls into distress, she can support herself easily, even in a foreign country, by means of her knowledge of these arts*

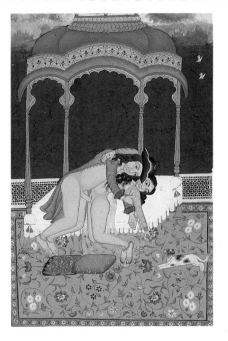

*The outer room, balmy with perfumes, should contain a bed, soft, agreeable to the sight, covered with a clean white cloth... having garlands and bunches of flowers upon it and a canopy above it, and two pillows...*

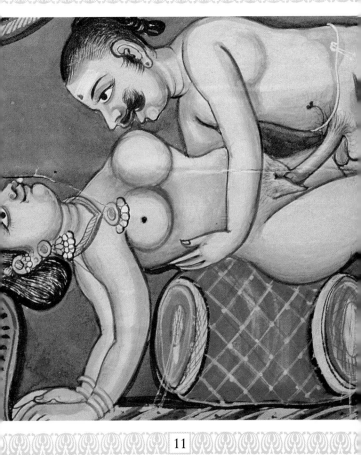

*Women being of a tender nature want tender beginnings... But he who neglects a girl thinking she is too bashful is despised by her as a beast ignorant of the working of the female mind*

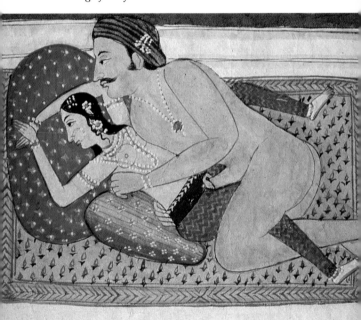

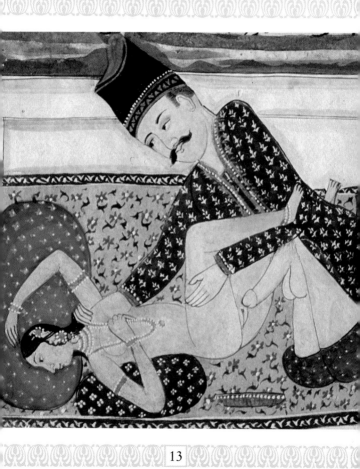

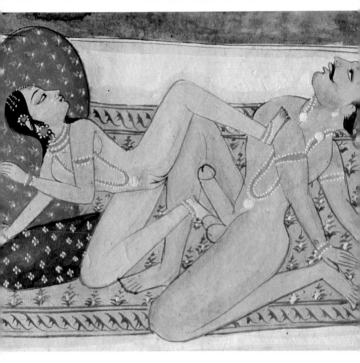

*The consciousness of pleasure in men and women is different... a man thinks 'This woman is united with me' and a woman thinks 'I am united with this man'*

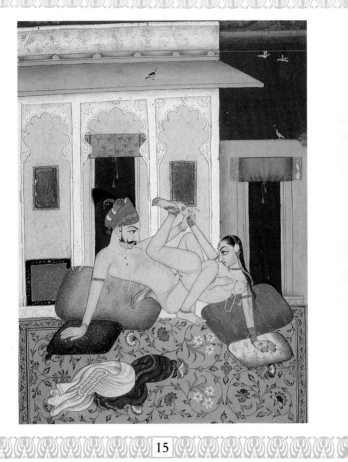

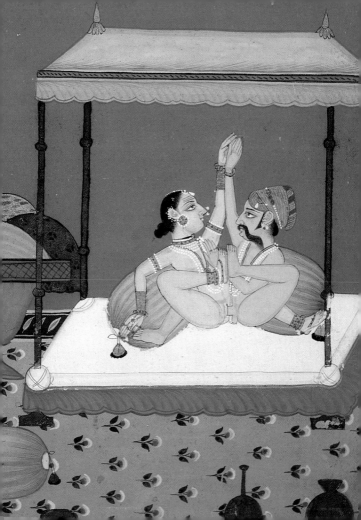

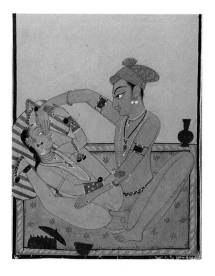

*At the time of meeting four kinds of embrace are used:
the twining of a creeper; the climbing of a tree; the
mixture of sesamum seed with rice; and the milk and
water embrace... the last two take place at the time of
sexual union*

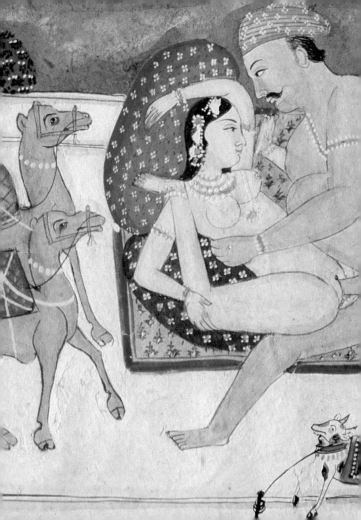

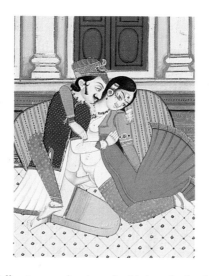

*The following are the places for kissing: the forehead, the eyes, the cheeks, the throat, the bosom, the breasts, the lips... if one of them touches the teeth, the tongue and the palate of the other, with his or her tongue, it is called 'the fighting of the tongue'*

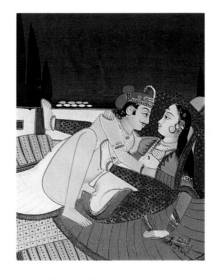

## THE WIFE OF INDRA

*When she places her thighs with her legs doubled... it is called the position of Indrani, and this is learnt only by practice*

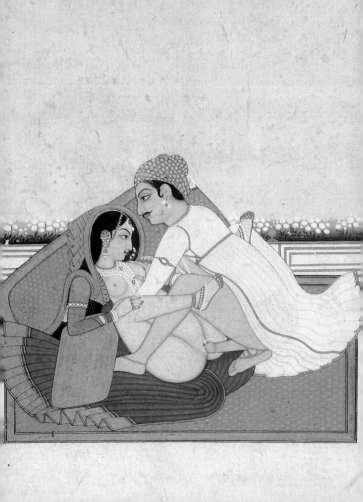

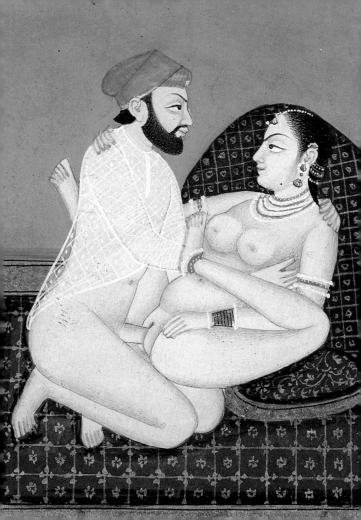

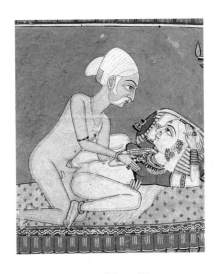

## VIJHRIMBITAKA - THE YAWNING

*When her lover kneels between her thighs and the
woman raises both her legs, opening them very wide...
it is called the yawning position*

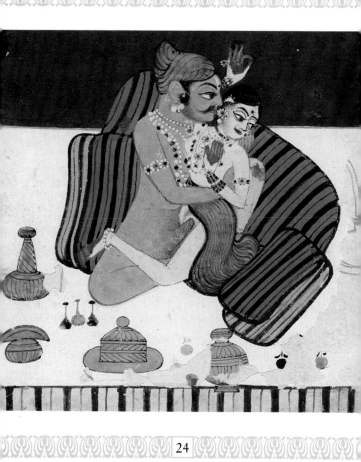

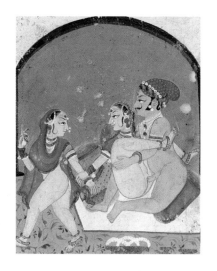

## THE MARE'S TRICK

*When she grips and milks her lover's lingam with her*
*yoni - as a mare holds a stallion - it is* Vadavaka,
*the Mare*

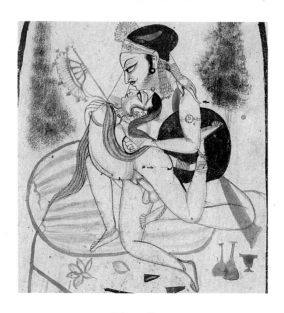

## THE COBRA

*If, lying with her face turned away, the fawn-eyed girl*
*offers you her buttocks and your penis enters the house*
*of love, this is* Nagabandha, *the coupling of the Cobra*

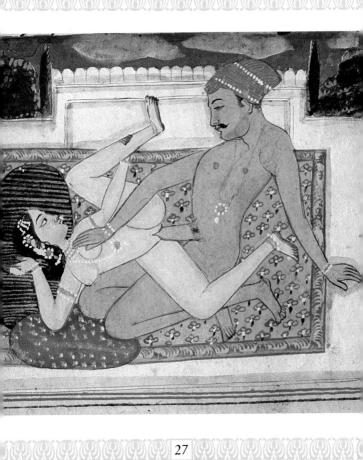

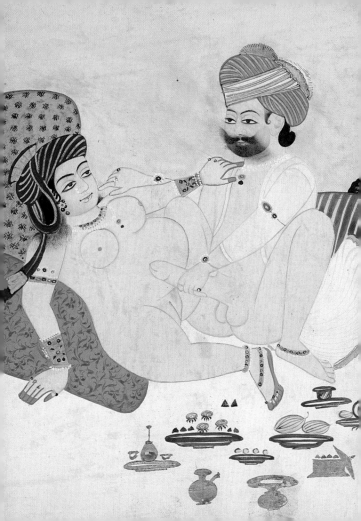

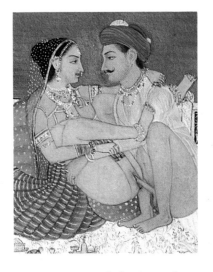

*Such passionate actions... which arise on the spur of the moment, and during sexual intercourse, cannot be defined and are as irregular as dreams*

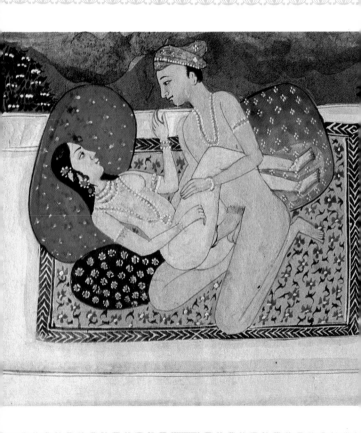

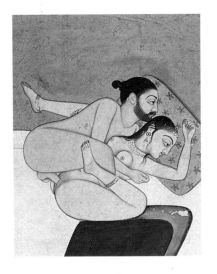

## THE CONCH

*When she lifts her thighs and you sit astraddle them,*
*your knees tightly clamped, kissing her tenderly and*
*riding saddle upon her buttocks, this is* Shankha,
*the Conch*

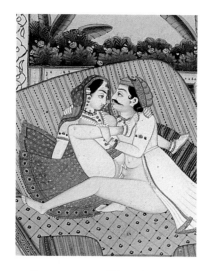

## PRENKHA - THE SWING

*In the pleasure room, decorated with flowers... they may also talk suggestively of things which would be considered as coarse, and not to be mentioned generally in society*

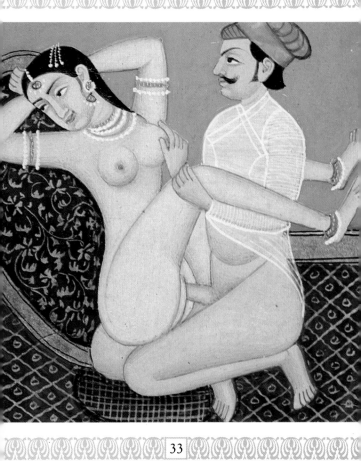

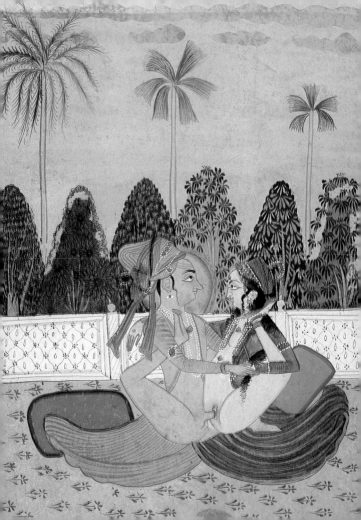

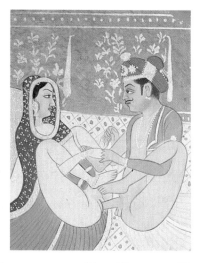

## BANDHURA - THE CURVED KNOT

*... if men and women act according to each other's liking, their love for each other will not be lessened even in one hundred years*

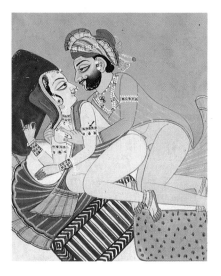

## THE DOG

*An ingenious person should multiply the kinds of congress after the fashion of the different kinds of beasts and birds... these generate love, friendship and respect in the hearts of women*

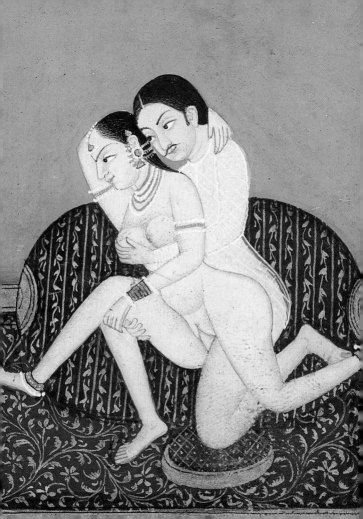

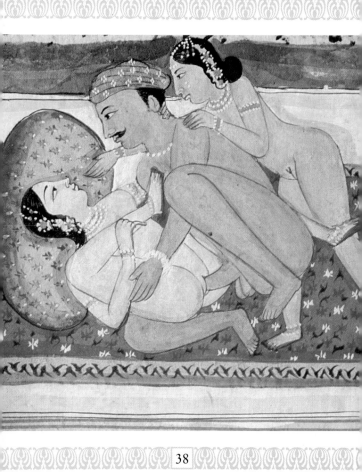

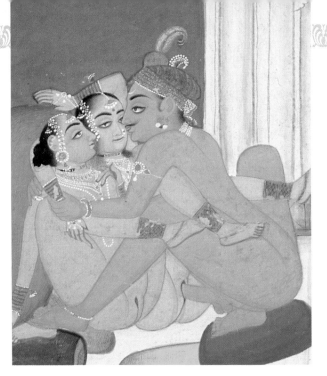

## THE UNITED

*When a man enjoys two women at the same time, both of whom love him equally, it is called 'the congress of a herd of cows'*

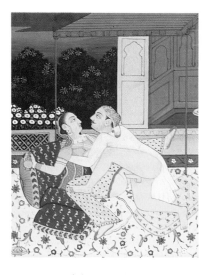

## THE PESTLE

*Stretched out like a pole in the middle of the bed, she
lies joined to you in lovemaking, her breathless cries
mounting as you polish the jewel of her clitoris: this is*
Mausala, *the Pestle*

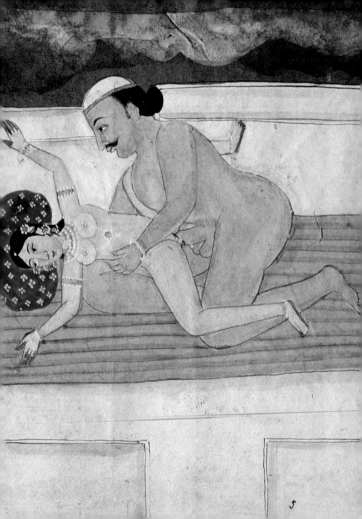

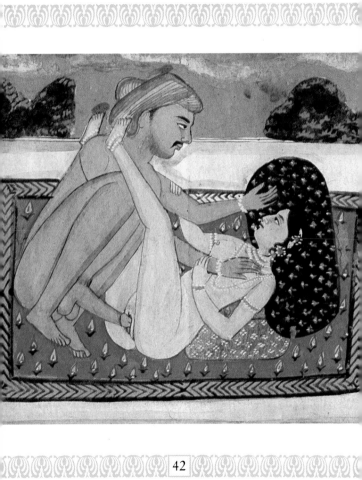

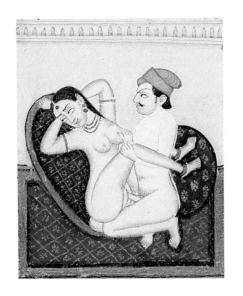

## UTPHULLAKA - THE FLOWER

*In this position, when the lingam is in the yoni, and is moved up and down frequently, and without being taken out, it is called 'the sporting of a sparrow'*

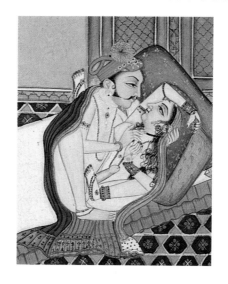

## CHURNING CURDS

*Caging your lover in your arms, you part her knees
and sink into her, crushing her body to yours: this is
known as* Dadhyataka, *or Churning Curds*

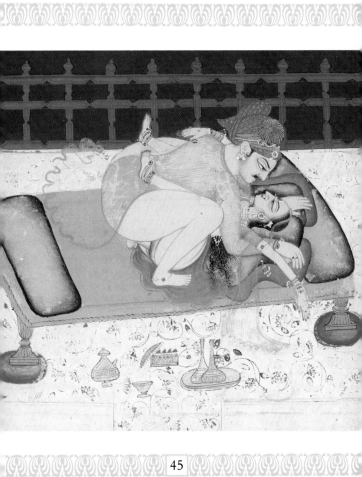

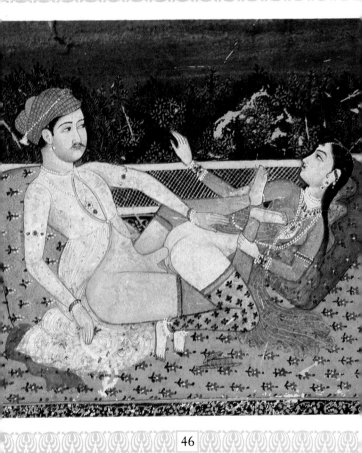

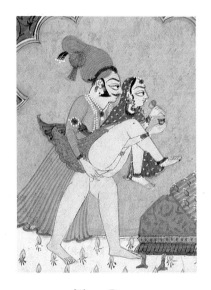

# THE DEER

*If your lustful lover buries her face in the pillow and goes on all fours like an animal and you rut upon her from behind as though you were a wild beast, this coupling is* Harina, *the Deer*

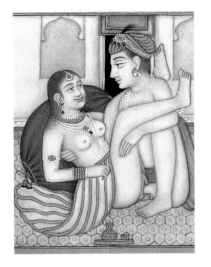

## *UTPIDITAKA – THE HIGH SQUEEZE*

*... a man should rub the yoni of a woman with his hand and fingers (as the elephant rubs anything with his trunk) before engaging in congress, until it is softened...*

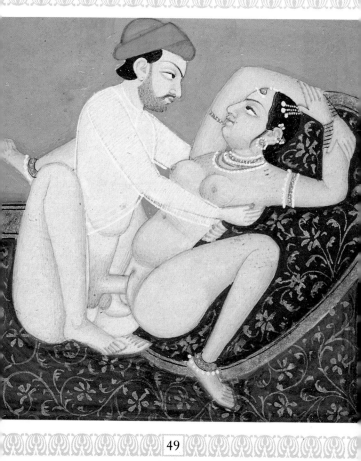

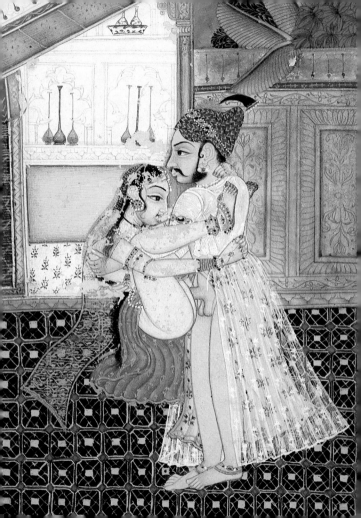

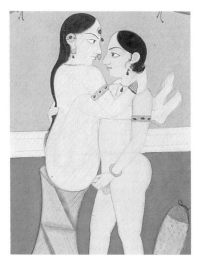

## THE KNEE-ELBOW

*If you lift the girl by passing your elbows under her knees and enjoy her as she hangs trembling with her arms garlanding your neck, it is called Janukurpura, the Knee-Elbow*

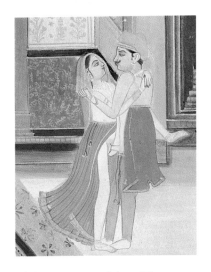

## *Tripadam – The Tripod*

*When a man and a woman support themselves on each other's bodies, or on a wall, or pillar, and thus while standing engage in congress, it is called 'the Supported Congress'*

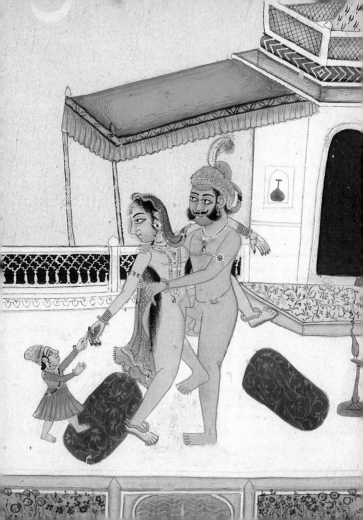

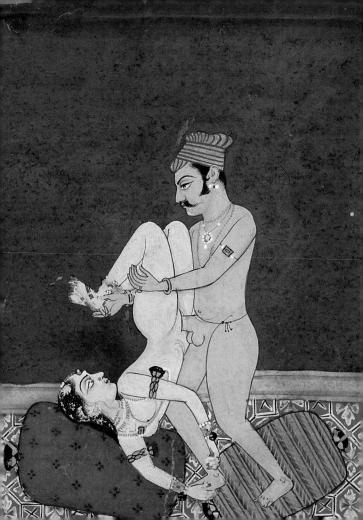

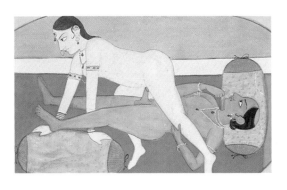

## VIPARITAKA (REVERSED)

*When the loving couple use their imagination to set the world upside down or when the woman plays the part of a man, these exciting games are Viparitaka or 'reversed congress'*

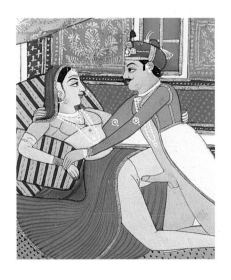

## GHATTITA - THE GRINDING

*While a man is doing to a woman what he likes best during congress, he should always make a point of pressing those parts of her body on which she turns her eyes*

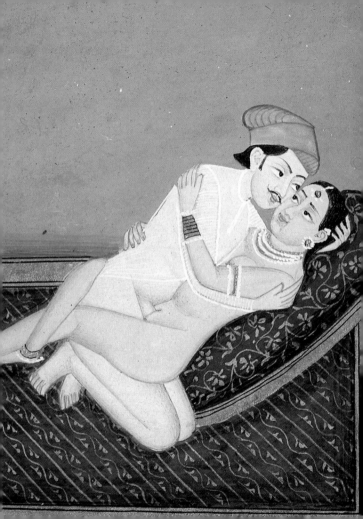

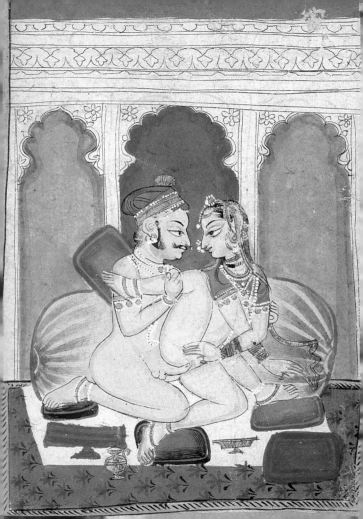

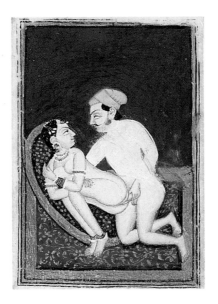

## HASTIKA - THE ELEPHANT

*In the same way can be carried on... the congress of a goat... the forcible mounting of an ass... the jump of a tiger... the rubbing of a boar, and the mounting of a horse*

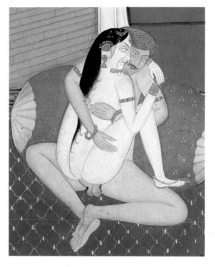

## THE BLACK BEE

*If you lie flat with your lover astride you, her feet drawn up and her hips revolving so that your lingam revolves deep within her sex, it is* Bhamara, *the Black Bee*

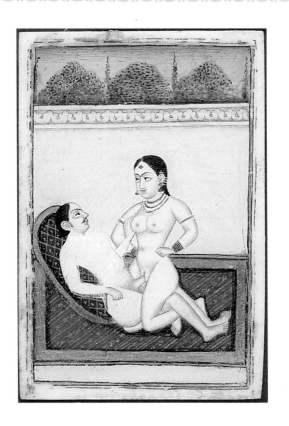

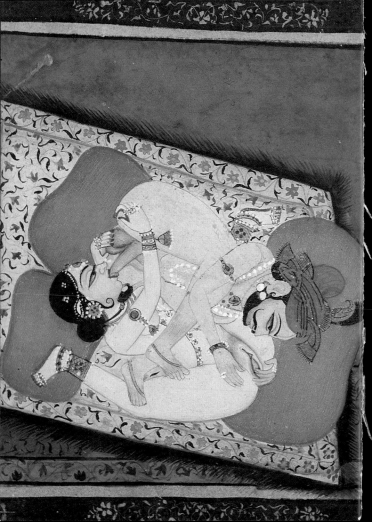

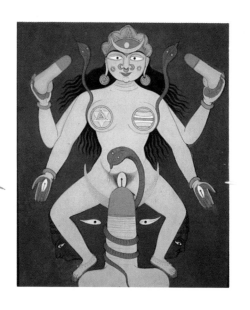

## KAKILA - THE CROW

*If, lying side by side, you simultaneously kiss each other's secret parts it is the lovemaking of the Crow... a sexual technique much practised by slaves, itinerants and other low persons*